You Are **NOT** Alone

Evelyn Evans – Gregg

You are NOT Alone
Copyright © 2016 by Evelyn Evans-Gregg
Kingdom Builders Publications

All rights reserved. No part of this book may be reproduced or transmitted in any form or by any means without written permission from the author.

ISBN:
Paperback: 978-0-692-72061-5

Photography – LH "Just Pose" Photography
Cover Designer – LoMar Designs

Editors:
Kingdom Builders Publications Editorial Staff
Carolyn Ash

Printed in USA
Go to this website for bookings and ordering:
www.kingdombuilderspublications.com

All Holy Scriptures are taken from the King James Version of the Bible unless otherwise stated.

DEDICATION

I dedicate this book to God, my Lord and Savior, who is head of my life.

To My Loving husband, Russell B. Gregg: who has been by my side continuously through sickness and in health.

To My Loving Daughter Meagan P. Gregg: who stood by me through it all, God was the rock through her as she was there for me.

In memory of my father, the late Willie Evans, my sisters the late Patricia A. Evans, and the late Judy Mouzon.

And to my loving family: Dr. Sandra L. Evans, whom has inspired and pushed me to keep writing, my mother JoAnn Evans, Gary F. (Linda) Evans, Corey N. Evans, Kimberly Mouzon, who was there for support through my illnesses.

To my extended family, all of the prayer worrier sisters in Christ, **Praising God in Spite of**. They are on the prayer line with me every Thursday night @ 9:00 pm CST and 10:00 pm EST. I thank all of you for your love and support. To God be the glory. He gets it all.

To Pastor T.W. and First Lady Patricia Campbell. Lady Campbell you are indeed a true friend, sister and prayer partner.

Love you all much.

Evelyn

CONTENTS

	Dedication	iii
	Acknowledgments	v
	Introductions	vi
1	Testimony	7
2	Stepping out on Faith	14
3	Walking by Faith Not by Sight	18
4	Being Tried by the Fire	22
5	Mustard Seed Faith	28
6	Seeking God's Face	32
7	Truth	36
	More About the Author	38

ACKNOWLEDGMENTS

To Minister Russell, Meagan Gregg, Vera Gregg, Veranda Orr, Gale Logan and Corey Evans for their financial contributions in bringing this book, **You Are Not Alone** into fruition.

INTRODUCTION

I have been through so much in my life and I have so much to be thankful for.

I wrote this book as a testimony to my life, and a guide to aid and bring comfort others who may be dealing with similar circumstances such as being alone, unforgiveness and living with a terminal illness.

Hopefully, my story will inspire others to stand for what they believe in and fight the good fight of faith, just as I did.

The past has taught me that people are consistent in being inconsistent, but my reaction to their actions is to have the love of God in my heart, walk it out in my life, forgive immediately; no matter what they do. With the love of God in your heart and life, *all things are possible.* **Philippians 4:13ᵇ**

TESTIMONY
Chapter One

My journey started the day I came into this world. At an early age, my parents had us in church. I'm the youngest daughter out of six siblings.

For as long as I could remember, we would go to the mourner's bench to receive Christ and be prayed over by the elders of the church. The Scripture **Romans 10:9** was embedded in our memory, *"If you confess with your mouth, Jesus is Lord, and believed in your heart God has raised Him from the dead, you will be saved."*

Before the age of 12, I was tender toward God and fascinated by His apparent presence. I accepted Him as my Lord and Savior. But it was a hush-hush affair in my heart because, in my upbringing, the fellowship where we attended, did not allow children to accept Jesus as Lord and Savior until 12 and older. We were taught that was unacceptable; possibly because it might be considered "playing with GOD."

Growing up, my siblings and I led a very

sheltered lifestyle. We only knew our world; not plundering outside our comfort zone, therefore we weren't altogether prepared for the real world. As lots of kids my age, I was naive about the happenings of the world, but to us, our childhood and teenage years seemed pretty normal and good.

I took the words of people at face value. I remembered what my Dad used to tell me, "Your word is all you have and if your word is no good then you are no good. Your word is your reputation." Those words were so important to me. I thought everyone had those values I was brought up on, but as it were, people don't always say what they mean, or mean what they say.

I am thankful for the wisdom of my dad. He gave us life's tidbits as we continued to grow up. My dad was much older than our mom, so he took the role as nurturer and disciplinarian. My dad taught me how to ride a bike, fly model airplanes, and fix on cars. I was blessed to have been brought up in a dual parent household. Dad and Mom raised us in Biblical principles, knowledge and wisdom. Although my dad is no longer with us, I know that he's in Heaven looking down on us all.

I am thankful for the power, grace and mercy of God and Him keeping me from dangers seen and unseen.

At the age of 25, my husband and I were married because we were very much in love. I later gave birth to our beautiful daughter. I bought into the American dream of marriage, the house with the white picket fence; boy was I disillusioned. It did not exist for me. I was fooled by the misconception of the world. Before my husband and I were married, I did not know he had a drug addiction because he kept it hidden for several years. Life didn't lend me the signs on anything I could grasp, seeing I was never exposed to that type of environment. When in my youth, the only drugs bad for you were alcohol, cigarettes, and marijuana.

My husband said to me a cold holiday morning, "The job needs me. I won't be gone long." This was a vivid memory of my daughter's second Christmas when he left for work and never returned. I stuck by him because I wanted to believe him and honor our wedding vows (*for better or worse, sickness and in health*), but the worse just kept getting worse and the sickness kept getting more pronounced. He was in and out of jail. The pastor asked me if I wanted him to get my husband out from our midst, but I defended him and told the preacher, no! I had grown tired of bailing him out every time he got into trouble; so I let him stay for a couple of days; that was my way of showing him tough love. We went to rehabilitation for drug abuse, Alcoholics Anonymous and Narcotics Anonymous (AA&NA) meetings with the 12 step program, we even tried church counseling. We would do fine for a while, then came the relapses and job losses.

This drug dependency was a clinical sickness. In the beginning, I kept on praying, going to church, falling on my face before the Lord, begging and pleading with the Lord to remove this stronghold Satan has put on my husband.

There was no denying, we were in trouble on every hand. We lost everything; our homes, cars, stability. Keeping up the pretense, we lived in a motel for six months and commuted back and forth from South Carolina to North Carolina.

I had reached that low and desolate place in my life. It didn't feel good I was not happy to be in this place, but it was all too familiar because I'd traveled this road and had been in and out of the low place so many times, but this time God granted an access to my very own room with God. I knew He was there in the dungeon with me. I recognize trouble comes to bring you to a place of dependence on the Creator. I was definitely having a valley crisis; everything was going wrong and there was no end. Thank God for His word that brought me comfort.

Psalms 119:11, *Thy word have I hid in mine heart, that I might not sin against God.*

That's when you have to remember the Scripture said *1I will lift up my eyes to the hills from whence comes my help. 2My help comes from the Lord. Who made the Heaven and Earth. 3He will not allow your foot to be moved: He who keeps you will not slumber. 4Behold, He who keeps Israel shall neither slumber nor sleeps. 5The Lord is your keeper: The Lord is your shade at your right hand. 6The sun shall never strike you by day: nor the moon by night. 7The Lord shall preserve you from all evil: He shall preserve your soul. 8The Lord shall preserve your going out and your coming in. From this time forth, and forevermore.* **Psalms 121:1: -8.**

God has seen me at my best and at my worst. He is always there helping us along the way;

carrying us when we couldn't carry ourselves: like the _Footprints in the Sand_.

I've seen my loved ones depart from this world of diseases like cancer, old age, septic poison of the blood, and brain tumors. I've seen and experienced the spirit of addiction tear our family apart numerous times. It appears he would take on more than he could handle and this would be a trigger for him to use, becoming self-absorbed by being over worked and not getting enough sleep. It was hard for him to find balance in life. We were always off kilter.

This spiritual behavior caused a lack of communication and family neglect as well as abandonment; something I experienced much too often.

According to the Scriptures, God is supposed to be first; then the spouse, family and job. Christ said "*Love your wife or husband as Christ loves the church*;" but instead of the Bible's picture, this is how it went; job, unhealthy recreational habits, mother-in-law. This was not spelled out in the vows.

So, here we go again.

She was blatantly disrespectful in my home. She had her way, and she vexed me every time she came to the breakfast table. Her son moved her in with us. Supposedly, it was to be only for two to three months at best, but it turned into a 24 month stay. I would occasionally speak to him about it, but in his defense and excuse not to change, he said I was trying to make him choose between his mother and me; which was, of course the farthest from the truth.

I became a stranger in my own home. His habits got him fired again and again, so he resorted to his personal comfort; doing drugs, which left us alone and him nowhere to be found.

Once again, I tried to hold on for him in his sickness, not knowing I was becoming a co-dependent as well as an enabler. My role was slowly disappearing. I became a walking, breathing, empty shell; invisible and nonexistent. My independence was gone. My identity and self-esteem had become nothing more than a dried up pea. Instead of being by my husband's side as his help mate supposed to, I was far in the distant shadows.

We constantly bumped heads. The Bible clearly speaks a man should cleave to his wife and become as one, but this did not happen. He cleaved to the other woman; his mother! I felt betrayed and denied in my own house, leaving me alone to care for our daughter and take care of his mother. That was wrong on every level.

I called his aunt telling her I was bringing her sister back home, because I wasn't able to afford to take care of her, my daughter, and myself.

STEPPING OUT ON FAITH
Chapter Two

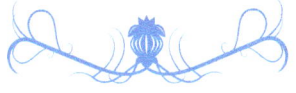

I know it was God keeping my daughter and me. She needed me and I needed her, and we both relied on God to keep us both. We lived there for about two years, just the two of us. It was one of the hardest situations I could have ever imagined for the two of us; probably harder for my daughter than for me. He has been in and out of our lives for 17 years, but through it all, God was there.

I thank you Lord for granting the desires of my heart.

I remember in the hottest of summer days, I would take my daughter down to South Carolina to my mother's house for the summer.

When I returned to N.C., I went on a manhunt. I had to save my husband; I had to save my marriage. I searched high and low for him; going through the drug infested neighborhoods, drug houses; all of this after getting off my job midnights. I even had some of the church members looking for him as well. Heard rumors he was renting the car for drugs, living in a drug house. We lost a total of 3 cars during Satan's trials of abandonment and temptations. It was rumored he was taking care of someone else's children and not his own. He had them thinking I put him out of the house and he didn't have a place to stay.

See the lie, but let the truth be told. He went to work and never returned; this is a drug addict's M.O. The Lord had allowed me to see the triggers, and the signs just before he would go out and use. He would start an argument for no apparent reason; acting very suspiciously, sleeping all the time, stealing things out of the house while I'm at work. I had the locks changed on the doors, but he still broke in. I couldn't take it anymore, so I moved.

My daughter and I moved into a 1-bed, 1-bath Apartment. This was something I could afford; the rent was only $375 monthly with water, and garbage included.

Sometime later, a house came available across the street a 3 bedroom 1 bath. My daughter was happy and so was I. She finally had her own room. That was clearly the happiest time for the both of us. We spent all weekend painting and decorating her room how she wanted it to be. I thank God for opening the doors for that 1bedroom apartment and the house across the street for us.

You see; we have the power and the authority to take back what the devil has stolen. Scripture said *"Satan comes to kill, steal and destroy."* The Lord said to Simon, *Satan has asked for you, he may sift you as wheat* as noted in **Luke 22:31**.

God had allowed me to recognize my enemy. I was sick and tired; and I had enough of the devil messing with my family. Satan was working my last nerve, and I was not going to let Satan win. My victory is in Christ Jesus. And *I can do all things through Jesus Christ, who strengthens me.* **Philippians 4:13**

One day I was reading a book by author Karl Payne, who wrote: *"In Christ we have the authority and the power to consistently walk above their temptations and propositions if we learn how to discern the source of our battles and apply the proper defense system God has designed for each enemy."* I, myself had to proclaim Spiritual Warfare on Satan himself. By putting on the hold armor of God, I was determined I was not going to let my husband be lost to drugs and alcohol; the traditional curses had to be broken. I declare and decree Satan would not; shall not destroy my family. Through my prayers and studying the word of God, He heard my cry and I continue to fight spiritually for my husband and my family, by never taken off my armor. Because as soon as you do, the enemy is there to destroy you through any means necessary. In The Name Jesus.

It was God whom allowed me to go into those drugs infused places and streets and not be harmed. He placed a hedged bush of protection all around me, by not letting no harm come to me.

I was walking by faith and not by sight.
2 Corinthians 5:7
Order my steps in thy word: and let not any iniquity have dominion over me. **Psalms: 119:133**.

He was with me leading and guiding me all the way with the Holy Spirit in the mist of it all. And where I found him, that's where the Lord told me to leave him. After finding him, we went through a dating process.

We dated for about 6 months while praying and asking the Lord if I should allow him to come back into our lives. I was hoping and praying this would be the last time our family would have to go through this unruly thing anymore. During this time, my daughter didn't know what was going on because I protected her from her father's ugly truth. My daughter's super hero, my groom was a practicing drug addict.

I prayed that God would deliver him from this temptation, because I knew it could be done. God can deliver you from any and all temptations you may have, if you so desire. Deliverance depends on how badly you want to be delivered from your temptations. Scripture said, *"If you delight yourself in him he would give you the desires of your heart."* **Psalms 37:4**. Our daughter loves the company of her dad, and now he's gone again. This time his job transferred him to S.C. to open up a restaurant. He knew this transfer was going to be permanent. But he allowed me to believe it was only temporary and he would be coming back after the opening of the store.

WALKING BY FAITH; NOT BY SIGHT
Chapter Three

As I approached my 39th birthday, I saw the instability in my family happening repeatedly, but this time it came with a twist, breast cancer; the Big "C."

When I received the news the first time, I was very distraught. Doctors told me I needed to get my affairs in order and I did, because the treatment I was going to receive was a very aggressive treatment. In my mind, I remembered what a dear friend told me that all sickness is not unto death. Sometimes we go through the fire, but when we come out, we don't smell like smoke.

Just like the three Hebrew boys: Shadrach, Meshach, and Abednego. Daniel 3:25

I was diagnosed December 2005. I was scheduled for surgery the first part of January of 2006. In March, I started chemotherapy along with blood thinner shots everyday which developed deep vein thrombosis in my legs, and in June I started 33 weeks of radiation. When I spoke with the radiologist, my hormone levels were at 40, which were considered high, but everything else was ok.

The type of breast cancer I had was called DCIS (Ductal Carcinoma-in-Situ). These are abnormal cells that evolve only in the ducts of the breast. The cells have not spread outside of the ducts of the tissues in the breast.

My daughter was with me, caring for me throughout my sickness. I was finally finished with all of my treatments, and my daughter was finished with school for the summer.

My husband came back to N.C. and moved us to S.C. February 2007, we were a family until he left us again in March. History has a way of repeating itself, when you make the wrong choices in life, or if you don't make what is wrong, right. Rock bottom came to my husband, and that affected us in a major way. Like Saul, on the road to Damascus, the bottom fell out for a change to take place with my husband.

"Then he fell to the ground, and heard a voice saying to him, "Saul, Saul, why are you persecuting Me?" **Acts 9:4**

I was blessed to move with my daughter to Florence. I knew in every situation God offers a way out.

Flee also youthful lusts: but pursue righteousness, faith, love, peace with those who call on the Lord out of a pure heart.
2 Timothy 2:22

We resided in Florence a little more than five years. I went back to work and school. My daughter was able to skip the 11th grade and graduated from high school with an honor cord a year early.

God has a way of dealing with us on His terms when we are disobedient or fall out of the will of God. In our sin we know that; sin is trying to get out of life what God did not put in it. God had put me in a place where I could not run and rescue him like I've always done. I could no longer be an enabler. I had to take my hands off of him and let God deal with his child.

It was called tough love. And by doing so, it allowed God to begin a work in his life. He had to be sifted as wheat by God and in doing so, he had to die to his fleshly desires on a daily basis.

He had to do this by not allowing himself to give into the desires of the flesh: eyes, ears, nose, and mouth. He had to learn a new focus; not giving in to those things that are not pleasing to the will of God. My husband was learning a new resolve; he who's in Christ Jesus is a new creature and all old things have passed away.

I believe God had answered my prayers; my husband and I have been reunited. It took 5 years of separation, while commuting from Florence to Columbia, and praying to God to make him a Godly man; to mature him into the man he would have Him be, not just what I wanted him to be. I've tried and it did not work on my own.
Remembering each night, as I fell to my face prostrate before the Lord; thanking God for my trials and my tribulations for bringing me through.

1Thessalonians: 5:16-18.
16Rejoice always, 17Pray without ceasing, 18In everything give thanks, for this is the will of God in Christ Jesus for you.

I continued praying to God that He would give me the ability to become stronger in Him during these trials, not only for myself but for my daughter. Not once did I give up on him, because God never gave up on me.

Hebrews 13:5
He will never leave you, nor will he forsake you.

I dug in deep and I was not going to let go until Satan was defeated. My family was back together the way God had ordained it. It was similar to being like Jacob in *Genesis 32:26. And he said: Let me go, for the day breaketh, and he said: I will not let thee go, except thou bless me.* I wasn't going to let go or give up until Satan gave back what he tried to take from me. Because: Satan has no power, and no authority.

TRIED BY FIRE
Chapter Four

Several years later, at 45 years old, for the second time, I was re-diagnosed with breast cancer July 19, 2011. The only difference was I had my husband for support this time around. The first time I was diagnosed with breast cancer, it was a burden to carry with just my daughter and me. She was in the 8th grade. I know taking care of me was a big responsibility for her, but she stuck right on in there with me.

I was very sick with pain throughout my body, nausea and the vomiting, weakness, and mouth sores. At times, it seems like the only way I was able to rest was on the cool of the floor with a waste paper basket by my head. The bed could not provide comfort during my time of sickness. I held on and made it through, because of God's grace and His mercy. We are overcomers and survivors of cancer, because our strength comes from the Lord.

Proverbs 14:26 *In the fear of the Lord, there is strong confidence, and his children will have a place of* *refuge.*

I still cry sometimes when I think about the struggles my daughter and I went through. Many times I felt like giving up, but God continued to remind me I needed to stay around a little while longer. My daughter and my husband needed me and I needed them. I thank God every day for what He is doing in my life. He continues to draw me closer to him through my prayers, my praise, my worship, and my studies with Him.

This time, it's in my right breast; same condition as the last time, but on the opposite side. Doctors and surgeons suggested I have a bi-lateral mastectomy (the removal of both breasts) with reconstructive surgery. I went through the chemotherapy and Herceptin infusion instead of the radiation treatment.

I felt like the poison was killing my mind, my body and my spirit for the second time. I was emotionally and physically drained from the inside out.

I remember putting on a mask to prove to my family and the world, "Hey, I've got this cancer all under control. I'm a fighter and I can beat this the second time around." When in actuality it doesn't matter how many times an individual goes through an illness, the body reacts differently. Being diagnosed with breast cancer for the second time was even harder to cope with than the first. The feeling of tiredness, vulnerability and depression came to the point I would actually start to cry.

Proverbs 19:23, *The fear of the LORD leads to life, And he who has it will abide in satisfaction; He will not be visited with evil.*

I would stay in bed for days at a time, not wanting to get up. I just wanted to pull the covers over my head and for it all to just go away. My mind and body were tired and confused; just sick of being sick every single day. I was sick all the time, with weakness and pain throughout my body with the chemotherapy. The treatment of chemo and Herceptin caused my body to be fatigued with muscle stiffness, my knees hurt all the time. I had an x-ray done on my knees; the x-rays showed I had deterioration of the bones in my knees.

I did not want to go through treatment for the second time or third time; NO MORE!

I finished my treatment for 2011, 2012 for the second breast cancer I had in 2011. I have closed the second chapter in my life. Now I have opened a third chapter in my life, for treatment of bone cancer.

I've tried physical therapy, it helped a little, but at the end of the day when everything comes to a head, my knees still hurt and even more when climbing up stairs. As I finished my treatments for the second time, I just knew something was just still not right. I knew what I was feeling in my chest was not right. The Holy Spirit allowed me to be in tune with my body. I was persistent with the doctor to have a PET/CT scan done, which is an imaging of the whole body. On July 2012, I found out through the biopsy taken showed the breast cancer had metastasized itself to the bone on the sternum of my chest.

We were all hopeful but the treatment did not perform as expected, The Doctor did not understand why the cancer did not respond to the treatment of the chemotherapy. We decided to get a second opinion from the Medical University of South Carolina (MUSC) in Charleston, SC. We needed options, and my husband and I were hopeful MUSC could be that place!

Being tried by fire for the third time, I sought solace through the Scriptures. There's an old cliché that says, "God is not going to put more on you, than what you can handle or bear."

Now I am facing secondary metastases of bone cancer. Doctors recommended an oral chemotherapy treatment along with hormone therapy, however there is no guarantee this treatment will work to slow down the progression.

It is not a cure, only a treatment, so to speak. This drug may have an effect for three to six months and the cancer may come back.

I started this medication in September 2012, and I've been on the medication for about five months and it has stopped the progression of the cancer. Thank God for working through the doctors and the medication for the stabilization of the cancer in my body.

It's February 2013, and I have to do 20 treatments of radiation, which is five weeks of treatments, which was one day out of the week. I was so thankful to God I didn't have to go through the full treatment. God has given me a sense of peace as I continue to go forward with the treatments. I remembered a song by my favorite singer Marvin Winans "I Feel Like Going On." God alone is giving me the endurance to GO ON!

After a year of being treated with chemotherapy and radiation, I was given another treatment of hormone blocker for a year to isolate the cancer in that area. In September 2014, I started the first round of chemotherapy for the fourth re-occurrence of cancer that had spread to the lymph node in my neck. This treatment is every 3 weeks in hopes of shrinking and fading away. I've had three treatments since then and every side effect is different, but there is one thing that remains constant; the nausea, vomiting, dry mouth, tiredness, hair loss, and weight gain always accompanied each chemotherapy treatment.

As I walk by faith and not by sight, the journey is becoming easier and easier. I'm not believing in what I see, nor encounter in the physical, but what I experience in the Spiritual. I am continuously being renewed in my heart and mind (*Ephesians 4:23*).

Proverbs 3:7-8. *Be not wise in thine own eyes: fear the Lord, and depart from evil. It shall be health to thy navel, and marrow to thy bones.*

I know as I continue to abide in the Lord, and His words abide in me, whatever I ask it shall be done in Jesus' Name. *(John 15:7).*

These Scriptures is where I have found my strength and my peace.

James 5:13-14
If any among you, are afflicted? Let him pray. Is any

merry? Let him sing psalms. Is anyone among you sick? Then he must call for the elders of the church and they are to pray over him, anointing him with oil in the name of our Lord.

Ephesians 4:23
And be renewed in the spirit of your mind.

Psalms 62:1-2
My soul finds rest in God alone: my salvation comes from him.
He alone is my rock and my salvation: he is my fortress; I will never be shaken.

Matthew 21:22
And all things, whatsoever ye shall ask in prayer, believing, ye shall receive.

MUSTARD SEED FAITH
Chapter Five

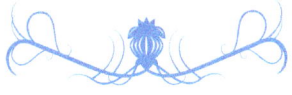

I prayed to the Lord; He brought me through the first, second and the third times, and He'll bring me through the fourth time; in fact, His record says I win EVERY TIME.

I asked the Lord: "Why do I have to go through this again for the fourth time?" In my prayer, I did not understand God's plan for me. He has given me through the Holy Spirit the gift of faith. This gift is to encourage and build me up in my most holy faith, then it builds up the Church through the confidence of God, and when you have the gift of faith, you trust that He is Sovereign, and He is good, and you put the full weight of your life in His hands. This I have done.

He is head of my life; for He is the Lord, my first priority, even before my day gets started. I'm thanking and giving Him praise for all He has done and is doing in my life.

I will always believe and trust in God. I know He

would never bring me to this place, if He couldn't bring me through this. With faith in God, I continued to stand on the promise God gave to Abraham. I believe His word is true. By faith we were saved and *Isaiah 53:5, by his stripes we were healed.*

I know God is in the mist of it all, even when my body is in pain every day, I'm still holding on. God is still keeping me. I continue to rest in God for my peace, safety, and comfort.

I even cry sometimes when I have to take insulin shots for the diabetes in my body, and for chemo treatments I have to take for a year. I cry but, I go through anyway.

Jesus cried out when He was in the garden of Gethsemane. In our cries, God hears us. When we are in our secret closet and wailing before the Lord, He hears us. When our hearts are pure and we worship Him in Spirit and in truth, He hears us; even when our hearts are burdened, and heavy laden, He hears us. He's all knowing and all seeing, all hearing, He is there.

Sometimes we have to take a moral inventory. This

means you are evaluating your motives; examining who you really are in Christ. God is continuously conforming us so we may be transformed to walk in His will and His ways.

Romans 12:2
Be not conformed to this world: but be ye transformed by the renewing of your mind, ye may prove what is good and acceptable and is the perfect will of God.

One thing I have learned when taking a spiritual inventory asking myself this important question: What characteristics do I display?

1. The one I exhibit. (the flesh of man)
2. The one I think I have. (the soul of man)
3. The one I truly have. (the human spirit of man)

In order to fulfil your spiritual inventory, you should follow these guidelines:

a. Make time-schedule time to be with the Lord,

Job 33:33 *"Be silent, and I will teach you wisdom."*

b. We must open our heart wide to see the real truth; trust God to give you the strength and courage you need.
c. Believe in God, when He created the

Heavens, and Earth and the creation of man, it was good.
d. By trusting in Him you can pray:

Dear Lord, you know my past, all the good and the bad things I've done. I ask you give me the strength and the courage to face the truth: and in doing so, help me to reach others you have placed along the way. Lord, I thank you for providing balance in my life. In Jesus' Name. Amen

Jeremiah 29:11

11 For I know the plans I have for you," declares the LORD, "plans to prosper you and not to harm you, plans to give you hope and a future.

Your hope and future is in Christ Jesus, and there will be times you don't know what to pray. This is when you submit yourself, allow the Spirit of the Lord to come into your heart, mind, body and soul, then He will direct your path because our steps have already been ordered by God.

We cannot be selfish, but we must surrender daily by asking God for help in our time of need. We can't fight this battle alone for if we try, we as people will mess it up.

We have to pray to the Lord, (as the elders say take it to the altar and leave it there) take your hands off of it because God doesn't need our help. He can handle the situation better than we can. He will give you serenity in the mist of your storm. He gives a kind of peace that surpasses all understanding.

Others will wonder how your deliverance came to pass? It's only because God is in it. You will have the victory in your life. God will have the glory because He deserves it!

SEEKING GOD'S FACE
Chapter Six

Psalms: 139:23-24;
Ps: 23, Search me, O God, and know my heart; test me and know my anxious thoughts.
Ps: 24, See if there is any offensive way in me, and lead me in the way everlasting.
Isaiah 1:18
Come now, let us reason together," says the Lord. "Though your sins are like scarlet, they shall be as white as snow, though they are red as scarlet, they shall be like wool."

My spirit is full of faith, but in my body, I wrestled. My human spirit prays my honest: "*Lord, if you're not going to take this sickness away, then please give me the strength to endure, give me the same strength that was given to Job to walk through his trials and tribulations; while giving God the glory.*"

Being honest with my Jesus led me to a place of strength and power. While getting closer to God, never fainting nor wavering, I stood firm, being like a tree planted by the river of ever flowing waters, being steadfast, unmovable, always abiding in the works of the Lord, being free to dance before Him, just like David, being free to worship, praise, and shout unto the Lord with a voice of triumph.

Unfortunately, bad things sometimes happen to good people. Because we were born into sin, we are all sinners. Job was the only one who was found faultless. I remembered how Job reacted when he was talking and walking with God. He complained about the trials of his tribulation, even when his wife and friends wanted him to either curse or repent to God. Job stood firm with them and denied their offer.

(paraphrasing)

Job said "I have done nothing wrong and I am not about to start now." Job 2:9 17:4-6. Although, Job was asking:

Why? God was asking: Who? God, even went into detail as to ask Job "Where were you, when I laid the foundation for all creation" Job 38:4:31, 39:26. Even towards the end when Satan thought he had the last say so, God was still there. After Job realizes he was nothing as he sits in dust and ash in repentance for everything was said. Job 42:6. In Job's obedience to God, God blessed Job with a double portion, giving Job 140 years, double the size of his heard as well as his children. Job was blessed beyond measure.

There is a Job in all of us, but when God allows Satan to sift us, we must stand firm and trust that God will do what we ask of Him. We can be blessed just like Job. I thank God for allowing me to see another day and be surrounded by people whose hearts are pure and love the Lord as much as I do.

I've learned to trust in the Lord more and more each day.

Psalms 46:1-2

God is our refuge and strength, a very present help in trouble.
Therefore, will not we fear, though the earth be removed, and though the mountains be carried into the midst of the sea.
Even Paul had a thorn in his side.

2 Corinthians 12-7:8:9:10

To keep me from being conceited because of all these surpassingly great revelations, there was given me a thorn in my flesh, a messenger of Satan, to torment me.
Three times I pleaded with the Lord to take it away

*from me. But the Lord said to me
"My grace is sufficient for you, for my power is made perfect in weakness."
Therefore, I will boast all the more gladly about my weaknesses, so Christ's power may rest in me.
For Christ's sake, I delight in weaknesses, insults, in hardship, in persecutions, in difficulties. FOR WHEN I AM WEAK, THEN I AM STRONG.*

I know God has elevated me to a Paul-like spirituality, where I have suffered because of the thorn in my flesh; the BIG "C." By faith, I am walking with Christ. Even though the Doctors cannot understand the miracle that has taken place in my body, God has allowed the medicine to work for the cancer in my bones to stop spreading. God left behind scar tissue that showed signs of healing.

Six months ago the Doctor told me I would die from Cancer. Probably so, but I know for now, my God is not through with me yet. He is a living God, a healing God, a miracle working God, and showing signs of wonders God. He continues to show Himself strong throughout my life and family's lives.

TRUTH
Chapter Seven

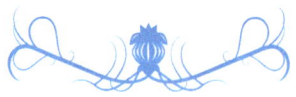

My faith walk with God has given me a Job experience, a Paul walk of faith with a thorn in my flesh, and an Abraham mountain top belief with a ram in the bush.

Now a Shadrach, Meshach and Abednego experience. I'm grateful even though I've been through the fire, I don't' smell like smoke, and I'm living a Hezekiah life, because God is not finished with me yet. God is still good to me. My life is a living testimony. When you see me, you wouldn't think of my life being the way it was. I'm so glad I don't look like my circumstances.

Everywhere the Lord is leading me, I'm telling my testimony of how awesome He is in my life. I continue to give Him all the glory and the praises of what He continues to do in my life.

Thank you Lord, for using my affliction to put me in touch with my need for You.

Psalms 73-26:28

My flesh and my heart may fail, but God is the strength of my heart and my portion forever.

But as for me, it is good to be near God. I have made the Sovereign Lord, my refuge. I will tell of all your good deeds.

I sit in amazement on how awesome God is just moving and working in my family's lives; my daughter has graduated from college with a degree in Music Business, Technology and is gainfully seeking her masters in Elementary Education, my husband is preaching and teaching the word of God. God has allowed him to graduate from college with a degree in pastoral ministries and Bible, and he's getting his masters in clinical counseling. Our marriage is stronger than it's ever been before, because God has strengthened the two of us through our trials. The power of prayer and the relationship we have with God continues to draw us closer to Him. God sustains me through this illness. The doctors say I have cancer, but cancer doesn't have me. He allows me to do what pleases him the most.

As I continue to write I hope someone out there will know, You Are Not Alone.

God is always with you. He will never leave you, nor will he forsake you.

MORE ABOUT THE AUTHOR

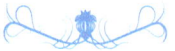

Evelyn Evans-Gregg is a native South Carolina, She the daughter of JoAnn Evans and the late Willie Evans of Florence S.C. She's married to Min. Russell Gregg for 23 years and they have a beautiful daughter named Meagan P. Gregg. Mrs. Gregg just finished writing the daily devotional readings for the June 2016, issue four, You Writers /LifeWay

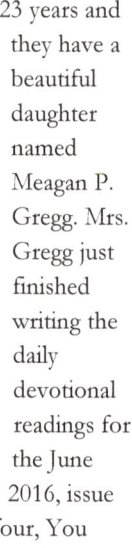

Resource and Publication. She just recently signed with Kingdom Builders Publications with CEO Louise Smith, for her first book titled **You Are Not Alone**. Mrs. Gregg enjoys Creative writing, refurbishing furniture, Home Interior/Floral Designed, singing praises unto the Lord with the praise team at her church, she serves as a deaconess, Chaplain on the Pastors Aide Ministry and also as one of the instructors for the New Members Orientation class as well as singing with a gospel group. She is a part of Praising God despite of Prayer Line that is on call every Thursday Night. Her gifts have allowed her to inspirer and encouraged those whom she meet.

www.ingramcontent.com/pod-product-compliance
Lightning Source LLC
Chambersburg PA
CBHW062106290426
44110CB00022B/2729